THE COMPLETE DASH DIET COOKBOOK FOR BEGINNERS

A Culinary Guide for Managing Blood Pressure with Nutrient-Rich Recipes, Proven Meal Plans, and Essential Tips for a healthy Lifestyle

George Evelyn

Table of content

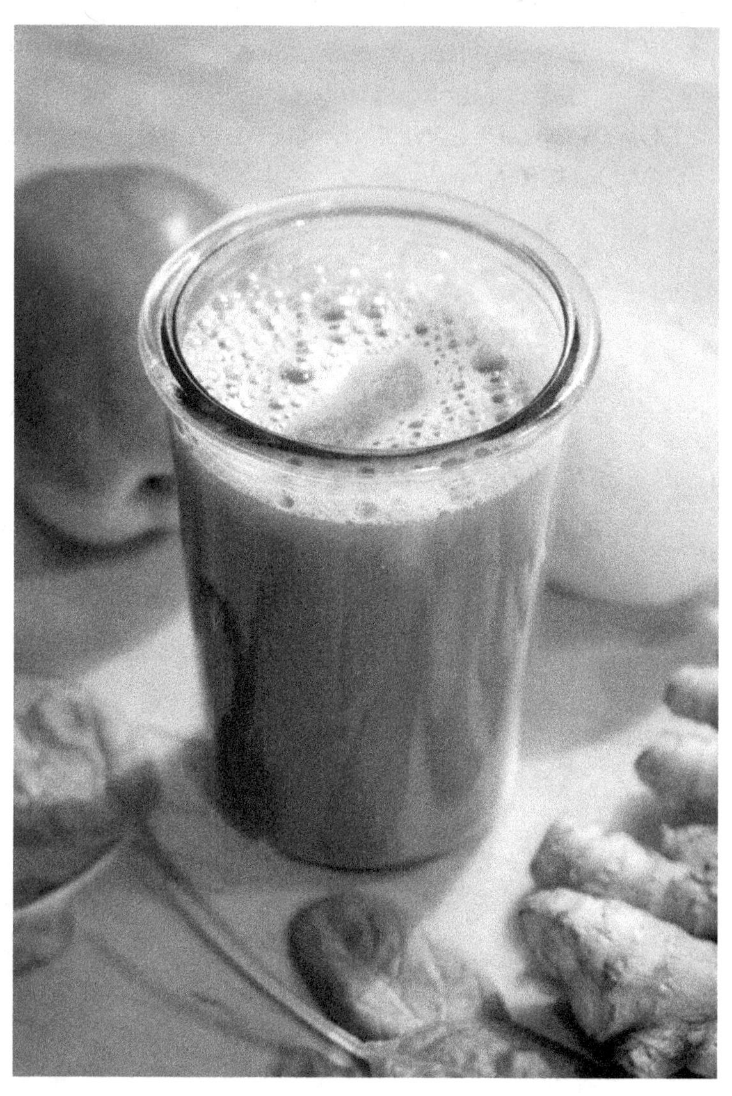

INTRODUCTION

The Complete DASH Diet Cookbook for Beginners is thoughtfully designed to provide an accessible entry point into the Dietary Approaches to Stop Hypertension (DASH) lifestyle, ensuring that individuals new to this approach find it both simple and easy to adopt. The cookbook's tailored features focus on simplicity and ease of adoption, offering a comprehensive guide for beginners.

1. **Clear and Concise Instructions:** The cookbook prioritizes clarity in its instructions, breaking down each recipe into easy-to-follow steps. Beginners can navigate the cooking process effortlessly, building confidence in their culinary skills as they progress through the book.

2. **Accessible Ingredients:** Recognizing that beginners may not have an extensive pantry, the cookbook emphasizes readily available and common ingredients. This not only simplifies the shopping process but also encourages beginners to explore DASH-approved foods without the burden of searching for rare or exotic items.

3. **Nutritional Guidance:** Understanding the importance of nutritional awareness, the

cookbook provides valuable insights into the nutritional content of each recipe. This empowers beginners to make informed choices, promoting a deeper understanding of the DASH principles and their impact on overall health.

4. **Meal Planning Support:** Recognizing the challenges of meal planning, especially for those new to the DASH diet, the cookbook offers pre-planned meal ideas. This feature helps beginners structure their weekly meals effortlessly, reducing the stress associated with figuring out what to eat while adhering to DASH guidelines.

5. **Variety and Flexibility:** To keep the experience enjoyable, the cookbook incorporates a diverse range of recipes. This variety ensures that beginners won't feel limited or bored with their food choices, promoting long-term adherence to the DASH lifestyle. Additionally, the cookbook provides options for customization, allowing individuals to tailor recipes to their taste preferences.

6. **Educational Components:** Beyond just recipes, the cookbook includes educational sections explaining the core principles of the DASH diet. Beginners can grasp the

rationale behind the dietary recommendations, fostering a deeper commitment to healthier eating habits.

7. **Meal Prep Tips:** Acknowledging the time constraints of modern life, the cookbook integrates practical meal prep tips. This assists beginners in planning and preparing meals efficiently, reinforcing the idea that adopting the DASH diet can be seamlessly integrated into a busy lifestyle.

The Complete DASH Diet Cookbook for Beginners goes beyond being a collection of recipes; it serves as a holistic guide, addressing the unique needs and challenges that beginners face. By prioritizing simplicity, accessibility, and education, the cookbook empowers individuals to embark on their DASH journey with confidence and ease.

Understanding the DASH Diet

The DASH (Dietary Approaches to Stop Hypertension) Diet is a dietary plan designed to help prevent and manage hypertension. It emphasizes a balanced and heart-healthy approach to eating. The key principles include:

1. **Low Sodium Intake:** DASH encourages reducing sodium intake to help control blood pressure. This involves limiting high-sodium foods like processed foods, canned goods, and salty snacks.

2. **Rich in Fruits and Vegetables:** The diet promotes a high consumption of fruits and vegetables, which are excellent sources of essential vitamins, minerals, and antioxidants. These foods contribute to overall health and help lower blood pressure.

3. **Lean Proteins:** DASH encourages lean protein sources such as poultry, fish, and plant-based proteins like beans and nuts. These choices provide necessary nutrients without excessive saturated fats.

4. **Whole Grains:** Whole grains are a significant component of the DASH Diet, offering fiber, vitamins, and minerals. This includes whole wheat, brown rice, oats, and quinoa.

5. **Dairy:** Low-fat or fat-free dairy products are recommended to ensure adequate calcium intake without excess saturated fats. This includes milk, yogurt, and cheese.

6. **Nuts, Seeds, and Legumes:** These are
    encouraged in moderation as they provide
    healthy fats, protein, and essential nutrients.

7. **Limited Sweets and Added Sugars:** The
    DASH Diet suggests minimizing the intake
    of sweets and added sugars. This helps
    maintain a healthy weight and reduces the
    risk of heart-related conditions.

8. **Moderate Alcohol Consumption:** If you
    consume alcohol, it should be done in
    moderation. Men are allowed up to two
    drinks each day, while women are limited to
    one drink.

Benefits of Adopting the DASH Diet

The DASH (Dietary Approaches to Stop
Hypertension) diet is a well-regarded eating plan
designed to reduce and prevent hypertension, but
its benefits extend beyond cardiovascular health.
Here's a comprehensive look at the advantages of
adopting the DASH diet:

1   **Blood Pressure Management:**
- The primary focus of the DASH diet is to lower blood pressure, making it an effective tool in preventing hypertension.
- Emphasis on potassium-rich foods, such as fruits and vegetables, helps balance sodium levels, contributing to blood pressure regulation.

2   **Heart Health:**
- By promoting a diet high in fruits, vegetables, and whole grains, the DASH diet supports heart health by reducing the risk of heart disease and stroke.
- Lowering cholesterol levels is another positive outcome, thanks to the diet's emphasis on low-fat dairy and lean protein sources.

3   **Weight Management:**
- The DASH diet encourages the consumption of nutrient-dense, lower-calorie foods, contributing to weight loss or weight maintenance.
- The inclusion of fiber-rich foods helps control hunger and promotes a feeling of fullness, supporting weight management goals.

4   **Bone Health:**
  - Adequate calcium and magnesium intake, promoted by the DASH diet, supports bone health, reducing the risk of osteoporosis.
  - Dairy products, nuts, and seeds included in the diet contribute essential nutrients for maintaining strong and healthy bones.

5   **Diabetes Management:**
  - The DASH diet can be beneficial for individuals with diabetes as it emphasizes whole, unprocessed foods, and limits refined sugars and carbohydrates.
  - The balanced macronutrient profile of the diet helps regulate blood sugar levels, making it a valuable component of diabetes management.

6   **Improved Nutrient Intake:**
  - The DASH diet encourages a diverse and nutrient-dense food intake, ensuring individuals receive a broad spectrum of essential vitamins and minerals.
  - Increased consumption of fruits, vegetables, and whole grains provides antioxidants, fiber, and various micronutrients.

7   **Reduced Sodium Intake:**
  - By focusing on whole foods and minimizing processed and high-sodium foods, the DASH diet helps individuals reduce their overall sodium intake.

- Lowering sodium intake is crucial for blood pressure management and overall cardiovascular health.

8   **`Lifestyle Adaptability`:**
- The DASH diet is adaptable and can be customized to individual preferences, making it sustainable for long-term adherence.
- Flexibility in food choices allows for a more realistic and achievable approach to healthy eating.

Chapter One

GETTING STARTED

Essential Kitchen Tools

To prepare DASH-friendly meals, it's essential to have the right kitchen tools and utensils that promote a heart-healthy and balanced diet. Here's a comprehensive guide:

1. **Cutting Board:**

   - Choose a sturdy, non-slip cutting board for chopping fruits, vegetables, and lean meats.

2. **Chef's Knife:**

   - Invest in a high-quality chef's knife to make precise cuts and streamline meal preparation.

3. Vegetable Peeler:

- Opt for a peeler to easily remove skins from vegetables, promoting a higher intake of fiber-rich produce.

4. Measuring Cups and Spoons:

- Ensure accurate portion control and adherence to DASH diet recommendations with proper measuring tools.

5. Food Scale:

- A scale helps monitor ingredient quantities, particularly for proteins and grains, supporting portion moderation.

6. Non-Stick Pans:

- Use non-stick cookware to minimize the need for excessive oil, aligning with the DASH diet's low-fat principles.

7. Steamer Basket:

- Steam vegetables to retain their nutrients, promoting a diet rich in potassium and other essential minerals.

8. Baking Sheets:

- Ideal for roasting vegetables or preparing lean proteins with minimal added fats.

9. Blender:

- Make heart-healthy smoothies or soups by incorporating a powerful blender for fruits and vegetables.

10.   Food Processor:

- Efficiently chop, slice, and dice ingredients, saving time in meal preparation.

11.   Garlic Press:

- Enhance flavor without excessive salt by incorporating fresh herbs and garlic using a press.

12.   **Salad Spinner:**

- Ensure crisp and fresh salads with a spinner to remove excess water from washed greens.

13.   **Mandoline Slicer:**

- Achieve uniform slices for vegetables, maintaining consistency in portion sizes.

14.   **Citrus Juicer:**

- Extract fresh citrus juice to add flavor to dishes without relying on salt.

15.   **Silicone Spatulas and Utensils:**

- Use heat-resistant silicone utensils to prevent scratching non-stick surfaces while cooking.

16.   **Colander:**

- Rinse canned goods to reduce sodium content, particularly for beans and vegetables.

17. **Glass Storage Containers:**

- Store leftovers and meal prepped items in glass containers to avoid chemical leaching from plastics.

18. **Nut Chopper:**

- Easily incorporate heart-healthy nuts into meals for added texture and nutritional value.

Grocery Shopping Guide

1 **Meal Planning:**

- Plan your meals for the week, incorporating DASH Diet principles of balanced nutrients and limited sodium.
- Create a weekly menu to guide your grocery list, ensuring variety and adherence to the DASH Diet.

2 **Fresh Produce:**

- Prioritize a colorful array of fruits and vegetables, aiming for at least 4-5 servings daily.

- Include leafy greens, berries, citrus fruits,
  and cruciferous vegetables for a diverse
  range of vitamins, minerals, and
  antioxidants.

3 Lean Proteins:

- Choose lean protein sources such tofu,
  skinless chicken, fish, beans, and lentils.
- Choose fatty fish like salmon for omega-3
  fatty acids, supporting heart health.

4 Whole Grains:

- Fill your cart with whole grains like quinoa,
  brown rice, oats, and whole wheat products.
- Look for whole grain options to increase
  fiber intake, aiding in digestion and
  promoting satiety.

5 Dairy or Dairy Alternatives:

- Choose dairy products like cheese, yogurt,
  and milk that are low in fat or fat free.
- Consider dairy alternatives such as almond
  or soy milk, ensuring they are fortified with
  calcium and vitamin D.

6   **Nuts and Seeds:**

- Add a range of nuts and seeds, including
  flaxseeds, chia seeds, walnuts, and
  almonds.
- These provide healthy fats, fiber, and
  essential nutrients, complementing the
  DASH Diet.

7   **Healthy Oils:**

- Choose heart-healthy oils like olive oil or
  canola oil for cooking and salads.
- Use these in moderation to meet dietary fat
  needs while maintaining a DASH-friendly
  approach.

8   **Herbs and Spices:**

- Stock up on a variety of herbs and spices to
  enhance flavors without relying on
  excessive salt.
- Experiment with herbs like basil, thyme, and
  spices like turmeric to add depth to your
  meals.

9   **Limit Processed Foods:**

- Minimize processed and packaged foods
  high in sodium, added sugars, and
  unhealthy fats.

- Read labels carefully, opting for products with minimal additives and preservatives.

10   Healthy Snack Options:

- Select healthy snacks like nuts, seeds, and fresh fruits. Avert processed snacks that are heavy in sugar and salt. Having nutritious snacks on hand supports the DASH Diet's focus on nutrient-dense eating.

11   Low-Sodium Choices:

- Be mindful of sodium content, opting for low-sodium or no-salt-added versions of canned goods and condiments.
- Rely on herbs, spices, and natural flavors to season your meals instead of excessive salt.

12   Hydration:

- Prioritize water as your main beverage to stay hydrated without added sugars or calories.
- Limit sugary drinks and be cautious of high-calorie beverages that may not align with the DASH Diet.

Meal Planning Tips

Step 1:

Set Caloric Goals
- Determine your daily caloric needs based on factors like age, gender, weight, and activity level. Make sure your consumption of the three macronutrients—fats, proteins, and carbohydrates—is balanced.

Step 2:

Prioritize Fruits and Vegetables
- Make fruits and vegetables the foundation of your meals. Aim for 4–5 servings of each per day, ensuring a colorful variety to maximize nutritional benefits.

Step 3:

Include Whole Grains
- Choose whole grains over refined ones. Incorporate foods like whole wheat, brown rice, oats, and quinoa for fiber, vitamins, and minerals.

Step 4:

`Opt for Lean Proteins`
- Give special attention to lean protein sources including lentils, fish, poultry, and tofu. Limit red meat intake and choose healthier cooking methods like grilling or baking.

Step 5:

`Incorporate Dairy or Dairy Alternatives`
- Include low-fat or fat-free dairy products or dairy alternatives. These supply vital nutrients, such as vitamin D and calcium.

Step 6:

`Emphasize Nuts, Seeds, and Legumes`
- Incorporate nuts, seeds, and legumes for healthy fats, protein, and fiber. These can be added to salads, yogurt, or enjoyed as snacks.

Step 7:

`Minimize Sodium Intake`
- Reduce sodium by choosing fresh, whole foods over processed options. Use herbs and spices for flavoring instead of salt, and

be mindful of condiments with high sodium content.

Step 8:

Choose Healthy Fats

- Incorporate foods high in healthful fats, such as fatty fish, avocados, and olive oil. These fats support heart health and provide essential nutrients.

Step 9:

Monitor Portion Sizes

- To control your calorie intake, pay attention to portion sizes. Use measuring tools or visual cues to avoid overeating and maintain a healthy weight.

Step 10:

Limit Added Sugars

- Reduce the amount of food and drink that has added sugar. Opt for natural sweeteners like honey or use fruits for sweetness.

Step 11:

Plan Balanced Meals and Snacks
- Design balanced meals that include a mix of all food groups. Plan healthy snacks like fresh fruit, yogurt, or raw vegetables with hummus.

Step 12:

Stay Hydrated
- Make sure you are properly hydrated by consuming a lot of water throughout the day. Limit sugary drinks and be mindful of caffeine intake.

Step 13:

Gradual Changes and Regular Monitoring
- Make changes gradually to allow for adjustment. Regularly monitor your progress, adjusting your meal plan as needed, and celebrate your successes along the way.

DASH Diet Sample Meal Plans

Breakfast:

1   **Greek Yogurt Parfait:**
    Layer Greek yogurt with fresh berries and a sprinkle of nuts for a protein-packed start.

2   **Oatmeal with Fruit:**
    Cook steel-cut oats and top with sliced bananas, berries, and a drizzle of honey.

3   **Vegetable Omelet:**
    Whip up an omelet with spinach, tomatoes, and bell peppers for a nutrient-rich breakfast.

4   **Whole Grain Pancakes:**
    Make pancakes using whole grain flour and top with yogurt and sliced peaches.

5   **Quinoa Breakfast Bowl:**
    Combine cooked quinoa with diced apples, cinnamon, and a dollop of low-fat Greek yogurt.

Lunch:

1 Grilled Chicken Salad:
Mix grilled chicken, leafy greens, cherry tomatoes, and a light vinaigrette.

2 Quinoa Salad:
Toss quinoa with cucumbers, feta cheese, olives, and cherry tomatoes for a satisfying salad.

3 Vegetarian Wrap:
Fill a whole-grain wrap with hummus, assorted veggies, and a sprinkle of seeds.

4 Salmon and Vegetable Stir-Fry:
Cook salmon with colorful vegetables and serve over brown rice or quinoa.

5 Turkey and Avocado Wrap:
Roll up lean turkey slices, avocado, and greens in a whole-grain tortilla.

Dinner:

1 Baked Cod with Lemon and Herbs:
Season cod with herbs and bake with lemon for a flavorful, low-fat dinner.

2 Vegetable Stir-Fry with Tofu:

Stir-fry tofu and a variety of vegetables in a
light soy-ginger sauce.

3   Lean Beef and Vegetable Skewers:
Skewer lean beef cubes with colorful bell
peppers and grill for a tasty meal.

4   Chickpea and Spinach Curry:
Simmer chickpeas and spinach in a flavorful
curry sauce, served with brown rice.

**5   Mushroom and Spinach Stuffed Chicken
Breast:**
Stuff chicken breasts with sautéed
mushrooms and spinach, then bake until
golden.

Snack Ideas:

1   Mixed Nuts and Seeds:
Combine almonds, walnuts, and pumpkin
seeds for a crunchy and nutritious snack.

2   Fresh Fruit Slices:
Enjoy a mix of apple, pear, and berries for a
refreshing snack.

3   Vegetable Sticks with Hummus:
Dip carrot, cucumber, and bell pepper sticks
in hummus for a satisfying crunch.

4   Yogurt with Berries:
Pair low-fat yogurt with fresh berries for a
quick and easy snack.

5   Whole Grain Crackers with Cheese:
Choose whole-grain crackers and pair them
with a serving of reduced-fat cheese.

Chapter Two

DELICIOUS MEALS

Breakfast Delights

Greek yogurt parfait with fresh berries and a sprinkle of nuts

A Greek yogurt parfait with fresh berries and a sprinkle of nuts is a delicious and nutritious dish that can be enjoyed for breakfast or as a healthy snack. To make this parfait, you will need nonfat plain Greek yogurt, fresh berries such as raspberries, blueberries, or strawberries, and a sprinkle of nuts such as almonds, walnuts, or granola. For added sweetness, you can also sprinkle some honey or maple syrup on top.

Here's a simple recipe for a Greek yogurt parfait with fresh berries and nuts:

Ingredients:

- 1 cup nonfat plain Greek yogurt

- ¼ cup fresh berries (raspberries, blueberries, or strawberries)
- ¼ cup sliced almonds, chopped walnuts, or granola
- 1 tablespoon honey or maple syrup (optional)

Instructions:

1. Blend sweetener with Greek yogurt if using in a small bowl until fully combined.
2. In a glass cup or mason jar, layer the Greek yogurt, fresh berries, and nuts or granola.
3. Repeat the layers as desired.
4. If desired, drizzle with maple syrup or honey.
5. Enjoy your delicious and healthy Greek yogurt parfait with fresh berries and nuts!

This parfait is a great source of protein, fiber, and healthy fats, making it a satisfying and wholesome meal or snack.

Whole grain toast with avocado

Whole grain toast with avocado is a simple and healthy breakfast or snack option that has gained popularity in recent years. The combination of crispy whole grain bread and creamy avocado creates a delightful contrast of textures and flavors.

Here's a comprehensive guide to making this delicious dish:

Ingredients

- 2 slices of whole grain or whole wheat bread, toasted until golden and crispy
- 1 ripe avocado, halved, pitted, and peeled
- 2 tablespoons chopped cilantro
- Juice of 1/2 lime
- 1/2 teaspoon red pepper flakes (optional)
- Salt and pepper to taste
- Optional toppings: fried, scrambled, or poached egg, tomatoes, bacon, beans, jalapeno, spinach, or salmon

Instructions

1. Toast the whole grain bread in a toaster until golden and crispy
2. In a small bowl, combine and mash the avocado, cilantro, lime, and salt and pepper to taste
3. Spread half of the avocado mixture on each slice of toasted bread
4. If desired, top with your choice of optional toppings, such as fried, scrambled, or poached eggs, tomatoes, bacon, beans, jalapeno, spinach, or salmon
5. Serve immediately and enjoy your delicious whole grain toast with avocado

- For the finest flavor and texture, use ripe avocados.
- Freshly squeezed lemon juice adds tartness and enhances the overall taste
- Olive oil adds a fruity, peppery flavor and a pleasant hint of sharpness
- Choose sturdy, thick-sliced whole grain bread for the best results
- Mash the avocado separately to avoid damaging the toast
- Feel free to experiment with different bread types, such as gluten-free bread for a gluten-free version

Oatmeal topped with sliced bananas and a drizzle of honey

Oatmeal topped with sliced bananas and a drizzle of honey is a delicious and easy-to-make breakfast option. Here's a comprehensive recipe to create this tasty dish:

Ingredients:

- 3/5 cup organic oats
- 1 1/2 cup oat milk (or low-fat milk)
- 2 Chiquita bananas

- 2 tbsp. walnuts and cinnamon (to serve)
- 2 tbsp. honey

Instructions:

1. Bring milk with oats to a boil over low heat. Simmer for approximately five minutes, stirring from time to time. Remove the pot from the stove and let it stand for 5 minutes to allow the oats to soak some more
2. Peel and slice the bananas
3. Add extra water or milk if the oatmeal is too thick.
4. Pour the oatmeal into a bowl or deep plate and spread the banana slices on top
5. Sprinkle with coarsely chopped walnuts and cinnamon
6. Add honey to taste

Spinach and feta omelet

A spinach and feta omelet is a delightful culinary creation that seamlessly blends the earthy goodness of spinach with the rich, tangy notes of feta cheese. This dish not only provides a burst of flavors but also offers a nutritional powerhouse, making it a fantastic choice for a wholesome breakfast or brunch.

Ingredients:

- **Eggs**: The foundation of the omelet, eggs provide a protein-rich base. For optimal results, use high-quality, fresh eggs.
- **Spinach**: Packed with vitamins, minerals, and antioxidants, spinach adds a vibrant green color and a nutritional boost to the omelet.
- **Feta Cheese**: Known for its crumbly texture and salty taste, feta cheese brings a creamy and tangy element, elevating the overall flavor profile.
- **Olive Oil**: Used for sautéing spinach, olive oil imparts a subtle richness and enhances the dish's Mediterranean flair.
- **Salt and Pepper**: Essential seasonings to enhance the taste of the eggs and balance the flavors.

Instructions:

1. **Prepare the Ingredients:**
   - Whisk eggs in a bowl and season with salt and pepper.
   - Wash and chop fresh spinach, ensuring it's free from any grit.
   - Crumble feta cheese for easy incorporation into the omelet.

2. **Sauté the Spinach:**
    - In a skillet over medium heat, warm the olive oil.
    - Sauté the spinach until wilted, releasing its moisture and concentrating its flavor.

3. **Mix and Cook:**
    - Combine the beaten eggs with the sautéed spinach, creating a vibrant, green mixture.
    - Sprinkle crumbled feta evenly over the egg-spinach mixture.

4. **Cook in a Skillet:**
    - Pour the mixture into a preheated skillet, allowing it to spread evenly.
    - As the edges set, gently lift them with a spatula to let the uncooked egg flow underneath, ensuring even cooking.

5. **Fold and Finish:**
    - Gently fold the omelet in half once it's mostly set but still a little runny on top.
    - Cook for a little longer until fully set but still moist, ensuring the feta melts slightly and the spinach retains its texture.

6. **Serve and Garnish:**
    - Slide the finished omelet onto a plate and garnish with fresh herbs like parsley or dill for added freshness.

Nutritional Highlights:

- Spinach is rich in iron, calcium, vitamins A and C, and various antioxidants.
- Eggs are a good source of necessary amino acids, high-quality protein, and a variety of vitamins.
- Feta cheese contributes calcium, phosphorus, and B vitamins.

Presentation:

Serve the spinach and feta omelet hot, perhaps alongside whole-grain toast, a side salad, or your favorite breakfast accompaniments.

Whole grain English muffin

Whole grain English muffins are a delicious and nutritious breakfast option that can be enjoyed in various ways. Here are some key aspects of whole grain English muffins:

Nutritional benefits

- **High in fiber**: Whole grain English muffins are a high-fiber, low-fat option compared to white flour alternatives, providing essential nutrients and a hearty flavor
- **Rich in nutrients**: They are made from whole wheat flour, which contains all the essential nutrients found in whole grains
- **Lower glycemic index**: Whole grain English muffins have a lower glycemic index compared to white flour, providing a slower release of energy and helping to maintain stable blood sugar levels

Ingredients

Common ingredients in whole grain English muffins include:

- Whole wheat flour
- Yeast
- Milk
- Unsalted butter
- Large egg
- Honey
- Cornmeal for dusting
- Some recipes may include additional spices like ground cinnamon or instant yeast

Preparation

1. Heat the milk and butter in a small saucepan until the butter has melted. Let the mixture cool until it is just warm, no hotter than 125°F
2. In the bowl of a stand mixer fitted with the dough hook, combine the milk, butter, egg, and honey
3. Once mixed, add the flour mixture and mix on low speed. Go to medium speed and knead for a full minute. Despite being moist and sticky, the dough should come together to form a ball.
4. Turn the dough out onto a floured work surface and roll it out to 3/4-inch thickness
5. Use a 3 1/2-inch round cutter to cut out English muffin shapes, re-re rolling the dough as needed
6. Place the dough rounds on a cornmeal-dusted baking sheet, cover with a towel, and let rise for 20 to 30 minutes, or until puffy
7. Preheat the oven to 325°F
8. Cook the muffins in a nonstick skillet or griddle over medium heat for 4 to 5 minutes on each side, or until they are crispy and brown.
9. Place the golden muffins back on the baking pan and bake for a further fifteen minutes.

Storage and freezing

Whole grain English muffins can be stored at room temperature in sealed plastic bags for up to two days or frozen for later use

Versatility
Whole grain English muffins can be used in various dishes, such as:
- Classic breakfast sandwiches
- Spread with butter or jam, or even made into little individual pizzas

spinach, banana, berries, and low-fat yogurt blended into a smoothie

A smoothie with spinach, banana, berries, and low-fat yogurt is a nutritious and delicious option for a quick meal or snack. Here's a comprehensive recipe for a blueberry banana spinach smoothie:

Ingredients:

- 1 cup spinach (fresh or frozen)
- 1/2 cup frozen blueberries or fresh
- 1/2 cup almond milk or milk of choice
- 1/2 cup yogurt (Greek or low-fat)
- 1 large ripe banana, peeled and cut up

- Optional: collagen powder, protein powder, or chia seeds for added nutrients and protein
- Optional: ice cubes for a thicker consistency

Instructions:

1. Gather all the ingredients.
2. Add the spinach, blueberries, yogurt, milk, banana, and any optional ingredients to a high-speed blender.
3. Blend until smooth and there are no bits of spinach left.
4. Taste the smoothie. Add extra milk or water if a thinner consistency is desired.
5. Pour the smoothie into glasses and serve immediately or refrigerate until ready to serve.

Whole grain toast with peanut butter

Whole grain toast with peanut butter is a nutritious and delicious option for breakfast or a snack. It offers a balanced intake of protein, carbs, and beneficial fats. Whole grain bread is a great source of fiber, which aids in digestion and helps keep you feeling full. Peanut butter offers protein and healthy fats, while the addition of banana slices provides essential nutrients like potassium. Here are a few variations of whole grain toast with peanut butter:

1. **Sprouted-Grain Toast with Peanut Butter & Banana**

   - **Ingredients:** 1 slice sprouted-grain bread, 1 tablespoon peanut butter, 1 medium banana, sliced

2. **Peanut Butter Banana Toast**

   - **Ingredients:** 2 slices whole wheat bread, 1 large ripe banana, 2 tablespoons honey, 1/4 cup peanut butter

3. **Peanut Butter Breakfast Toast 4 Ways**

   - This recipe offers different combinations of toppings for whole grain toast with peanut butter, providing variety and flavor

4. **Whole Wheat Toast with Peanut Butter and Banana**

   - This recipe suggests topping the toast with cinnamon and chia seeds for added flavor and nutrients

5. **Peanut Butter-Banana Cinnamon Toast**

- **Ingredients:** 1 slice whole-wheat bread, toasted, 1 tablespoon peanut butter, 1 small banana, sliced, Cinnamon, to taste

Lunchtime Favorites

Grilled chicken salad with mixed greens, cherry tomatoes, cucumbers, and a light olive oil dressing

Grilled Chicken Salad with mixed greens, cherry tomatoes, cucumbers, and a light olive oil dressing is a refreshing and nutritious dish that combines the flavors of Mediterranean cuisine. Here's an extensive recipe for this delicious salad:

Ingredients:

- Two cups of fresh mixed greens (lettuce of several varieties)
- 1 cucumber

- 1 bell pepper
- 3 cherry tomatoes
- 1 carrot
- 1 tbsp canned corn
- 50 g grilled chicken (breasts/file)
- Parmesan cheese
- 1 slice stale bread
- Balsamic vinegar
- Olive oil
- Lemon
- Salt and pepper to taste

Instructions:

1. Prepare the dressing by combining olive oil and balsamic vinegar in a 1:3 ratio. Squeeze in some water or lemon juice, a dash of salt, and a little pepper. Shake in a jar or thoroughly mix with a whisk until thoroughly blended.
2. Assemble the salad in a bowl. Place the washed salad greens, cucumber and bell pepper slices, halved cherry tomatoes, carrot sticks, and a tablespoon of canned corn. Add chicken bites and bread croutons
3. If you're not using pre-grilled chicken, season your chicken and put it in a hot pan to grill on both sides for a couple of minutes. Take off the heat, let cool, and then cut into smaller pieces.
4. Slice the stale bread into cubes and roast it in the pan for a few minutes.

5.   When toasted, set aside to cool
6.   Wash and drain the mixed greens. Use any variety of lettuce or a combination of them.
7.   Peel and slice the cucumber. Clean and cut your bell pepper (I had a kind in my garden that was light green).
8.   Add some shaved Parmesan cheese and the balsamic dressing to the salad.
9.   Serve immediately and enjoy your refreshing Grilled Chicken Salad with mixed greens, cherry tomatoes, cucumbers, and a light olive oil dressing.

Quinoa or brown rice on the side

Quinoa and brown rice are both versatile and nutritious side dishes that can be easily prepared and combined with various ingredients to create a variety of flavors. Here are some details on how to prepare these grains and their potential uses in different dishes:

Quinoa

- Quinoa is a gluten-free grain that provides fiber, protein, and minerals, supporting a healthy digestive system
- It cooks quickly and can be prepared in advance and stored in the refrigerator

- Quinoa can be used as a base for salads, pour-over meals, creamed soups, and stir-fries
- To cook quinoa, combine 1 cup of dry quinoa with 2 cups of water or broth in a saucepan, bring to a boil, reduce heat, and let it simmer for about 15-20 minutes until the water is absorbed

Brown Rice

- Brown rice is also a gluten-free grain that provides fiber, protein, and minerals, supporting a healthy digestive system
- A stovetop meal takes roughly forty minutes to prepare.
- Brown rice can be used as a base for various dishes, such as stuffed peppers, casseroles, and salads
- To cook brown rice, combine 1 cup of dry brown rice with 2 cups of water or broth in a saucepan, bring to a boil, reduce heat, and let it simmer for about 40 minutes until the water is absorbed

Quinoa and Brown Rice Combination

- Quinoa and brown rice can be cooked together in a pot with broth or separately and then mixed
- A Southwestern-style salad can be made with a combination of cooked brown rice,

quinoa, corn, black beans, bell pepper,
mango, and cilantro
- A healthy brown rice quinoa blend can be
  used as a side for meats or as a base for
  various dishes such as stir-fries and salads
- Parsley quinoa and brown rice pilaf is
  another delicious option, combining quinoa,
  brown rice, vegetable broth, parsley, and
  lemon zest

Vibrant Salad Creations

Vibrant Salad Creations is a term that refers to the creation of colorful, flavorful, and nutritious salads. These salads can be found in various recipes and culinary explorations, offering a wide range of options for healthy and delicious meals. Some key aspects of Vibrant Salad Creations include:

- **Variety**: Vibrant Salad Creations offer a diverse range of salads, from light and tangy mixes to hearty veggie-protein combos, catering to different tastes and dietary preferences

- **Seasonality**: Salads can be tailored to the seasons, with refreshing summer salads packed with vibrant fruits and vegetables, and hearty winter salads filled with warm and comforting ingredients

- **`Visual Appeal`**: The presentation of
  vibrant salads is often as important as their
  taste, with many recipes focusing on
  creating visually appealing and colorful
  dishes

- **`Culinary Journey`**: Vibrant Salad
  Creations can take you on a culinary
  journey, exploring various flavors, textures,
  and ingredients from around the world

- **`Health Benefits`**: Salads are a healthy
  choice for any meal, and vibrant salad
  creations can be packed with essential
  nutrients, vitamins, and minerals, making
  them a valuable addition to your diet

To create your own vibrant salad creations,
consider the following tips:

1. Choose fresh, high-quality ingredients with
   a variety of colors, textures, and flavors.
2. Experiment with different vegetables, fruits,
   nuts, and seeds to create unique and
   flavorful combinations.
3. Consider the season and your personal
   taste preferences when selecting
   ingredients and dressing.
4. Take the time to present your salad in an
   aesthetically pleasing manner, as visual

appeal can enhance the overall dining experience.

5. Experiment with different culinary techniques and recipes to find your own signature salad creations.

Whole grain tortilla wrap with turkey and vegetables

A Turkey and Vegetable Wrap with Whole Grain Tortilla is a nutritious and flavorful option that combines lean protein, fresh vegetables, and whole grains. The whole grain tortilla adds a boost of fiber and essential nutrients, contributing to a well-balanced meal.

Ingredients:

1. Whole Grain Tortilla: Choose a high-fiber tortilla for added nutritional benefits.
2. Turkey Breast: Opt for lean turkey breast slices as a protein source, which is lower in fat compared to other cuts.
3. Vegetables: Include a colorful variety such as lettuce, spinach, tomatoes, cucumbers, bell peppers, and any other favorite veggies for added vitamins and minerals.
4. Condiments: Add flavor with condiments like mustard, hummus, or a light vinaigrette.

These not only enhance taste but also provide healthy fats and additional nutrients.

Assembly:

1. Spread the Base: Lay the whole grain tortilla flat and spread a thin layer of your chosen condiment evenly across its surface.
2. Layer Turkey: Place the turkey breast slices on top of the tortilla, ensuring an even distribution for consistent flavor in each bite.
3. Vegetable Variety: Pile on a generous amount of fresh vegetables. This not only adds crunch and texture but also contributes essential vitamins and minerals to your wrap.
4. Wrap it Up: Carefully fold the sides of the tortilla towards the center and then roll it up tightly from the bottom, creating a secure wrap.

Nutritional Benefits:

1. Whole Grains: The whole grain tortilla provides complex carbohydrates, fiber, and various nutrients, promoting digestive health and providing sustained energy.
2. Lean Protein: Turkey breast is a lean protein source, aiding in muscle maintenance and repair without excessive fat intake.
3. Vitamins and Minerals: The assortment of vegetables delivers a range of vitamins,

such as A, C, and K, along with minerals like potassium and folate, supporting overall health.

Customization:

Feel free to customize your Turkey and Vegetable Wrap based on personal preferences and dietary needs. You can experiment with different vegetables, condiments, or even add a sprinkle of herbs or spices for extra flavor.

Mixed green salad with a balsamic vinaigrette

A mixed green salad with a balsamic vinaigrette is a simple and delicious side dish or light lunch option. The combination of fresh greens, tangy vinaigrette, and crunchy toppings creates a well-balanced and flavorful salad. Here's a recipe to make a mixed green salad with a balsamic vinaigrette:

Ingredients:

- 5 oz. bag of spring mix or greens
- 10 grape tomatoes
- ½ cucumber
- ¼ cup feta cheese

- 1 tbsp. olive oil
- ½ tbsp. balsamic vinegar
- 1 tbsp. lemon juice
- ¼ tsp. salt (or to taste)
- ¼ tsp. ground black pepper (or to taste)

Instructions:

1. In a small bowl, whisk together the olive oil, balsamic vinegar, lemon juice, salt, and black pepper to create the balsamic vinaigrette
2. Place the mixed greens, grape tomatoes, cucumber, and feta cheese in a serving bowl
3. Over the salad, drizzle with the balsamic vinaigrette and toss to mix.
4. You can also add your favorite nuts, seeds, or other toppings for extra crunch and flavor
5. Serve immediately.

Chickpeas, cherry tomatoes, and feta cheese in a quinoa salad

Quinoa salad with chickpeas, cherry tomatoes, and feta cheese is a delicious and nutritious dish that combines the powerhouse ingredients of quinoa, chickpeas, and cherry tomatoes. Here's a comprehensive recipe to make this tasty salad:

Ingredients:

- 1 cup uncooked quinoa
- 1 pint cherry tomatoes, halved
- 1/2 English cucumber, chopped
- 1 cup crumbled feta cheese
- 1 cup chickpeas, rinsed and drained
- 2/3 cup kalamata olives, halved and quartered
- 1/2 cup chopped red onion
- Greek dressing (optional)

Instructions:

1. Cook the quinoa according to package instructions.
2. While the quinoa is cooking, chop the cherry tomatoes, cucumber, red onion, and kalamata olives.
3. In a large bowl, combine the cooked quinoa, cherry tomatoes, cucumber, red onion, kalamata olives, and feta cheese.
4. If desired, drizzle the salad with Greek dressing or a lemon vinaigrette made from olive oil, lemon juice, garlic, Dijon mustard, salt, and pepper
5. Serve the salad warm, at room temperature, or cold.

Delectable Dinners

Baked salmon with lemon and herbs

Baked salmon with lemon and herbs is a simple and delicious dish that can be prepared in less than 30 minutes. The combination of lemon, herbs, and olive oil creates a flavorful and healthy meal that is perfect for a quick and satisfying dinner. Here's a step-by-step guide to making this dish:

Ingredients:

- 3-4 salmon filets
- 2 Tablespoons butter melted
- 2 medium lemons
- 1/4 cup finely chopped fresh herbs (basil, parsley, rosemary, or thyme work well)
- 3 cloves garlic minced
- kosher salt and black pepper

Instructions:

1. Preheat the oven to 425 degrees F. If your filets have skin, lay the salmon, skin-side down, on a parchment paper-lined baking sheet.
2. Evenly brush the filets' tops with the melted butter.

3. Juice one lemon, and slice the other into thin rounds. Arrange the lemon slices on top of the salmon.
4. In a small bowl, mix together the chopped herbs, garlic, salt, and black pepper. Drizzle the fish with the herb mixture.
5. Bake the salmon in the preheated oven for 12-15 minutes, or until the salmon is cooked to your desired level of doneness.

Steamed broccoli and carrots

Steamed broccoli and carrots is a simple and healthy dish that can be prepared in a few easy steps. Here's a comprehensive guide to preparing this nutritious side dish:

Ingredients:

- 1 cup broccoli florets
- 1/2 cup carrots, cut into bite-sized pieces or julienne cut
- 2 tablespoons lemon juice
- 1 teaspoon seasoned salt, or to taste

Instructions:

1. Prepare the vegetables: Cut the broccoli florets and carrots into bite-sized pieces or julienne cut the carrots
2. Steam the vegetables: Place a steamer basket in a large saucepan with 2 to 3 inches of water. Bring the water to a boil, then add the broccoli and carrots to the steamer basket. Cover and steam over medium heat for about 5-10 minutes until the vegetables are crisp-tender
3. Season and serve: Once the vegetables are tender, transfer them to a serving bowl. Add the lemon juice and seasoned salt, then toss gently to coat. You can also top the vegetables with butter and salt and pepper for extra flavor

Nutritional Information:

This dish is low in calories and high in essential nutrients. For example, a serving provides about 25.8 calories, 0.23g of fat, 5.83g of carbohydrates, 0.9g of fiber, and 1.39g of protein. It's also a good source of vitamins A and C, as well as potassium and calcium. Steaming is a healthy cooking method that helps retain the nutrients in the vegetables. This dish is not only quick and easy to prepare, but it also makes a colorful and nutritious addition to any meal. For a variation, you can also add other

seasonings such as garlic, herbs, or a sprinkle of
parmesan cheese to enhance the flavor of the dish

Mashed sweet potatoes

Mashed sweet potatoes are a popular side dish that
can be prepared in various ways, offering a
delicious and versatile alternative to traditional
mashed potatoes. Here are some key steps and
tips for making mashed sweet potatoes:

1. Ingredients: To make mashed sweet
   potatoes, you'll need sweet potatoes, butter,
   milk or cream, and salt and pepper to taste.
   You can also add other flavors, such as
   brown sugar, honey, or browned butter, to
   sweeten the dish. Some recipes also
   include additional spices like cinnamon or
   thyme for extra flavor

2. Cooking the sweet potatoes: Peel the sweet
   potatoes and dice them into large or small
   cubes. Boil the potatoes until tender, and
   then drain them well. Alternatively, you can
   bake sweet potatoes in the oven at 400°F
   for about 1 hour or until fork-tender

3. Mashing the sweet potatoes: Use a hand
   masher, hand mixer, or immersion blender
   to mash the cooked sweet potatoes. For a

chunkier texture, use a fork or hand masher, and for a smoother consistency, use a hand mixer or immersion blender

4. Adding flavor: After mashing, add warm milk or cream, and stir in butter and any additional sweeteners or seasonings to taste. Adjust the seasoning with salt and pepper as needed. Some recipes also suggest adding vanilla extract for extra flavor

5. Serving: Mashed sweet potatoes can be served hot, with additional butter or fresh herbs like thyme or cinnamon for garnish (optional). You can also make mashed sweet potatoes ahead of time and reheat them on the stovetop or in the microwave before serving

Stir-fried tofu with mixed vegetables

Stir-fried tofu with mixed vegetables is a delicious and nutritious meal option. Here's a comprehensive recipe to make this dish:

Ingredients:

- 1 lb extra-firm tofu

- 2.5 oz long beans or green beans
- 1 small carrot, diced
- Other vegetables of choice (e.g., peas, mushrooms, bell peppers, onions)
- 8-10 cloves garlic, roughly chopped or minced
- 1 tablespoon toasted sesame oil (or substitute with peanut or coconut oil)
- 1/4 cup low-sodium soy sauce (ensure gluten-free for GF eaters)
- 1 tablespoon fresh grated ginger
- 2 tablespoons organic brown sugar (reduce slightly for less sweet sauce)
- 1 tablespoon agave or maple syrup (or honey if not vegan; reduce slightly for less sweet sauce)
- 1 tablespoon cornstarch
- Optional: protein of choice (e.g., shrimp, diced chicken)

Instructions:

1. Press the tofu to remove excess moisture and cut it into small cubes. Set aside.
2. In a small bowl, whisk together soy sauce, ginger, brown sugar, agave, maple syrup, and cornstarch to create the sauce. Set aside.
3. A big wok or skillet should be heated to medium-high heat. Swirl in the sesame oil to coat.

4. Add the diced carrots and other vegetables to the skillet. Cook for 5-7 minutes, stirring often, until the vegetables have some color and have softened a bit.
5. Pour the sauce over the vegetables and stir to coat. Cook for another 3-5 minutes, stirring often, until the sauce has thickened.
6. Add the tofu to the skillet and stir to coat. Cook for another 3-5 minutes, stirring often, until the tofu is heated through and the sauce has thickened.
7. If desired, add your choice of protein (e.g., shrimp, diced chicken) and cook for an additional 1-2 minutes.
8. Remove from heat and serve immediately. Enjoy your stir-fried tofu with mixed vegetables over rice or on its own

Grilled shrimp with a lemon and garlic marinade

Grilled shrimp with a lemon and garlic marinade is a delicious and easy dish to prepare. To make this dish, you will need ingredients such as shrimp, salt, pepper, olive oil, lemon juice, garlic, red pepper flakes, and parsley. The shrimp can be marinated in a mixture of these ingredients for about 15-30 minutes before grilling. Once marinated, the shrimp can be grilled for 2-4 minutes on each side until they turn pink and opaque. The result is juicy and flavorful shrimp with a hint of citrus and garlic.

Here's a simple recipe for Lemon Garlic Grilled Shrimp:

Ingredients:

- 1 lb. shrimp, uncooked
- 1 teaspoon salt
- ½ teaspoon pepper
- 1/3 cup olive oil
- 2 Tablespoon lemon juice
- 1 Tablespoon garlic, minced
- ½ teaspoon red pepper flakes
- 1 tablespoon parsley, fresh & finely diced

Instructions:

1. In a bowl, mix the olive oil, lemon juice, minced garlic, red pepper flakes, salt, and pepper.
2. Toss the shrimp to coat after adding them to the bowl. Let it marinate for 15-30 minutes.
3. Preheat the grill to high heat. Thread the shrimp on skewers.
4. Grill the shrimp for 2-4 minutes on each side until they turn pink and opaque.
5. Sprinkle with fresh parsley and serve.

Roasted Brussels sprouts are a delicious and healthy side dish that can be prepared in under 30 minutes. They are crispy and tender, with a golden brown exterior and a flavorful interior. Here's a comprehensive guide on how to roast Brussels sprouts:

Ingredients:

- 1 1/2 pounds Brussels sprouts, trimmed and halved
- 3 tablespoons extra-virgin olive oil
- 3/4 teaspoon kosher salt
- 1/2 teaspoon freshly ground black pepper
- Optional flavor additions: balsamic vinegar, honey, lemon juice, zest, Parmesan, thyme leaves, red pepper flakes, nuts, or pepitas

Preparation:

1. Preheat the oven to 400°F (204°C) and place the oven rack in the middle position
2. Every Brussels sprout should have any yellow or broken leaves removed before being sliced in half lengthwise, from tip to clipped end.

Roasting:

- Arrange the Brussels sprouts in the middle of a sizable baking sheet with a rim.
- Drizzle with olive oil and sprinkle with salt, pepper, and any other desired spice additions
- Roast the Brussels sprouts for 20-25 minutes, until crisp and lightly charred on the outside and tender inside
- The exact timing may vary depending on the size of the sprouts

Seasoning and Serving:

- Optional: Toss the roasted Brussels sprouts with balsamic vinegar, honey, lemon juice, zest, Parmesan, thyme leaves, red pepper flakes, nuts, or pepitas for added flavor
- Serve the roasted Brussels sprouts as a side dish or incorporate them into a main course, such as a veggie frittata or breakfast casserole

Chapter Three

QUICK AND HEALTHY SNACKS

A spoonful of almond butter spread over some apple slices

Apple slices with a tablespoon of almond butter is a simple and nutritious snack that can be enjoyed by people of all ages. This delicious combination of crisp apple slices and creamy almond butter provides a variety of health benefits. Here are some key aspects of this tasty snack:

Ingredients

- 1 apple
- 1 tablespoon almond butter
- Optional toppings: sliced almonds, walnuts, dark chocolate chips, cinnamon, or seeds

Instructions

1. Slice the apple crosswise into thin slices
2. Spread each slice with almond butter

3. Top with your choice of optional toppings,
    such as sliced almonds, walnuts, dark
    chocolate chips, cinnamon, or seeds

Nutrition

- Apples are a good source of fiber and
  antioxidants
- Almond butter provides healthy fats,
  proteins, and minerals
- This snack is a good source of calcium and
  iron

Variations

- You can use other types of apples, such as
  Honeycrisp or Granny Smith, depending on
  your preference
- Instead of almond butter, you can use other
  nut butters like peanut or cashew butter
- For a added crunch, you can top the apple
  slices with granola or oatmeal

Serving Suggestions

- Enjoy the apple slices with almond butter as
  a snack or a light meal
- You can also pair it with plain Greek yogurt
  or oatmeal for a more substantial snack or
  breakfast

Carrot and celery sticks with hummus

Carrot and celery sticks with hummus is a healthy and delicious snack option that can be enjoyed as a mid-morning or afternoon snack. The combination of nutrient-dense and fiber-full carrot and celery sticks, along with the protein and fiber-rich hummus, makes for a satisfying and nutritious snack. Here's a simple recipe to make carrot and celery sticks with hummus:

Ingredients:

- Carrots and celery sticks (washed, hand-cut, and ready to grab and go)
- Hummus (store-bought or homemade)

Instructions:

1. Arrange the carrot and celery sticks on a serving platter or plate
2. In a food processor or blender, place cooked carrots and puree until smooth
3. Add hummus and cumin to the food processor or blender, and process until well blended
4. Refrigerate the hummus for 1 hour to blend the flavors

5. Serve the hummus as a dip for the carrot and celery sticks

Handful of unsalted nuts

A handful of unsalted nuts, approximately 30 grams or 1/3 of a cup, is a nutritious and beneficial snack that can be included in a balanced diet. Nuts are rich in unsaturated fats, protein, fiber, vitamins, and minerals, which contribute to overall health and well-being. Different types of nuts, such as almonds, Brazil nuts, cashews, hazelnuts, macadamias, pecans, pine nuts, pistachios, and walnuts, have similar nutrient content and can be included in a healthy diet

Health Benefits of Unsalted Nuts

1. `Heart Health`: Nuts contain protective antioxidants and are rich in monounsaturated and polyunsaturated fats, which can help lower bad cholesterol levels and reduce the risk of heart disease
2. `Weight Management`: Nuts are rich in fiber and healthy fats, which can help you feel fuller for longer and may aid in weight management
3. `Diabetes Prevention`: Nuts have a low glycemic index and can help regulate blood

sugar levels, making them a suitable snack for people with diabetes

4. **Immune Boost:** Nuts are a good source of vitamins A, C, and E, as well as minerals like folate, magnesium, zinc, copper, and selenium, which can help boost immunity and protect against various diseases

5. **Brain Health:** Nuts contain essential nutrients like omega-3 fatty acids, vitamin E, and antioxidants, which can support brain health and may help prevent cognitive decline

How to Include Nuts in Your Diet

- As part of a balanced diet, you can have a handful of raw or roasted unsalted nuts (around 30g or ¼ cup) per day.
- Nuts can be added to salads, yogurt, oatmeal, or smoothie bowls for added nutrition and texture
- Consider making nut butter or tahini (sesame paste) as a spread or dip for fruits, vegetables, or whole-grain crackers

Tips for Consuming Nuts

- Choose unsalted nuts to avoid the higher sodium content in salted nuts
- Roasting nuts enhances their flavor but has little impact on their fat content

- If you cannot tolerate the hard texture of nuts, consider eating them in unsweetened and unsalted paste forms such as nut butter and tahini

Nut and Seed Mixes

Nut and seed mixes are versatile and nutritious blends that combine various types of nuts and seeds, offering a tasty and wholesome snack option. These mixes typically include a variety of nuts such as almonds, walnuts, cashews, and peanuts, along with seeds like sunflower seeds, pumpkin seeds, and chia seeds.

Key Components:

1. **Almonds**: Rich in vitamin E and healthy fats, almonds provide a crunchy texture and a subtle sweetness to the mix.
2. **Walnuts**: Packed with omega-3 fatty acids, walnuts contribute a distinct flavor and additional nutritional benefits.
3. **Cashews**: Creamy and mild in taste, cashews add a delightful buttery element while providing essential minerals like zinc and magnesium.
4. **Peanuts**: A familiar favorite, peanuts offer protein and a satisfying crunch.

5. **Sunflower Seeds**: High in vitamin E, magnesium, and selenium, sunflower seeds contribute a nutty flavor and a nutritional boost.
6. **Pumpkin Seeds**: Also known as pepitas, these seeds are rich in iron, zinc, and magnesium, adding a chewy texture to the mix.
7. **Chia Seeds**: Packed with fiber and omega-3 fatty acids, chia seeds bring a nutritional punch and a gelatinous texture when hydrated.

Nutritional Benefits:

- **Protein**: Nuts and seeds are excellent plant-based protein sources, making the mix a satisfying snack that can help keep you fuller for longer.
- **Healthy Fats**: The inclusion of nuts provides monounsaturated and polyunsaturated fats, which are heart-healthy and support overall well-being.
- **Vitamins and Minerals**: These mixes are rich in essential nutrients like vitamin E, magnesium, zinc, and antioxidants, promoting various aspects of health.

Health Considerations:

- **Portion Control**: While nutrient-dense, nut and seed mixes are calorie-dense, so moderation is key.
- **Allergies**: Individuals with nut allergies should be cautious and opt for mixes that exclude allergens.
- **Salt and Sugar Content**: Some commercially available mixes may contain added salt or sugar, so it's advisable to check labels for a healthier option.

Versatility:
Beyond being a standalone snack, nut and seed mixes can be incorporated into various dishes such as yogurt parfaits, salads, or used as a topping for oatmeal. The mix of textures and flavors adds a delightful element to both sweet and savory recipes.

Fruit-Based Desserts

Fruit-based desserts are a versatile and delicious way to enjoy the natural sweetness of fruits. They can be made using a variety of fruits such as apples, pears, strawberries, peaches, blueberries, and more. Popular fruit-based desserts include:

1. **Crisps:** These desserts feature a mixture of fruits and a crumbly topping, often made with oats, flour, and butter. The combination of sweet and crunchy flavors creates a delightful contrast.

2. **Cakes:** Fruit-based cakes incorporate fruits into the cake batter, either as a puree, a mix-in, or as a topping. These cakes can be made with various fruits, such as apples, berries, or tropical fruits.

3. **Trifles:** Trifles are layered desserts that typically consist of a cake or sponge, fruit, and whipped cream or custard. The combination of textures and flavors creates a satisfying and elegant dessert.

4. **Pies:** Fruit pies are a classic dessert that features a pastry crust filled with fruits, often combined with sugar and spices. The filling can be made with various fruits, such as apples, berries, or peaches.

5. **Cobblers:** Cobblers are similar to pies but feature a biscuit or cake-like topping instead of a pastry crust. The topping is often sprinkled with sugar, which caramelizes during baking, adding a delicious crunch to the dessert.

6. **Cheesecakes:** Fruit-based cheesecakes incorporate fruits into the cheesecake batter, often as a puree or a mix-in. The combination of creamy cheese and sweet fruits creates a refreshing and indulgent dessert.

7. **No-Bake Desserts:** No-bake fruit desserts are perfect for those who prefer a quick and easy option. These desserts can be made without an oven and often require minimal preparation time. Examples include fruit salads, fruit bars, and fruit-topped desserts.

Chapter Four

DASH DIET FOR SPECIAL OCCASIONS

Celebratory Menus

Some celebratory menus for the DASH diet cookbook include:

Breakfast

1. **6-grain hot cereal**
   A warm and hearty breakfast option that is high in fiber and nutrients.
2. **Overnight oatmeal**
   A creamy and customizable breakfast option that can be made the night before for an easy and nutritious start to the day.

Lunch

1. **Asian pork tenderloin**

A flavorful and tender pork dish that
can be served with a variety of side
dishes.

2. **Turkey medallions with tomato salad**

A light and flavorful lunch or dinner
option that combines lean turkey
with a refreshing tomato salad.

Dinner

1. **Baba ghanoush**

A popular Middle Eastern dip made
from eggplant, tahini, and spices,
often served with pita bread or fresh
vegetables.

2. **tarragon, onion, and wild rice paired with baked chicken**

A delicious and healthy chicken dish
that combines the flavors of onion,
tarragon, and wild rice.

3. **Baked cod with lemon and herbs**

A simple and healthy fish dish that is
high in omega-3 fatty acids and can
be served with a variety of side
dishes.

Sides and Snacks

1. **Warm rice and pintos salad**

A versatile and colorful side dish or
main course that combines brown

rice, pintos, and a variety of fresh
vegetables.

2. **Raspberry peach puff pancake**
   A simple and satisfying treat that is
   perfect for brunch or dessert,
   offering a combination of fruity and
   sweet flavors.

3. **Grilled Southwestern steak salad**
   A hearty and flavorful salad that
   combines grilled steak, peppers,
   onions, and a variety of fresh
   vegetables.

Celebratory Occasions

For special occasions, consider the following DASH
diet recipes:

1. **Baked salmon with lemon and dill**
   A festive and flavorful fish dish that
   is high in omega-3 fatty acids and
   can be served with a variety of side
   dishes.

2. **Lentil chili**
   A hearty and flavorful vegetarian
   dish that is perfect for game day or
   family gatherings.

3. **Chocolate-chia pudding**
   A delicious and healthy dessert
   option that is low in sodium and high

in flavor, making it a great alternative to traditional chocolate treats.

MAINTENANCE AND BEYOND

Staying on Track

Staying on track with the Complete DASH Diet Cookbook for Beginners involves a combination of mindful meal planning, consistent adherence to DASH (Dietary Approaches to Stop Hypertension) principles, and establishing sustainable habits. Here's a comprehensive guide on how to stay on track:

1 Understanding the DASH Diet:

- Familiarize yourself with the core principles of the DASH diet, emphasizing whole foods rich in potassium, calcium, magnesium, and fiber.
- Be aware of recommended daily servings for different food groups, such as fruits, vegetables, whole grains, lean proteins, and dairy.

2 **Meal Planning:**

- Make a food plan in advance to guarantee a healthy, well-balanced diet.
- Incorporate a variety of DASH-friendly ingredients into your weekly meal plan, including fresh produce, lean proteins, and whole grains.
- Experiment with different cooking techniques to enhance flavors without compromising nutritional value.

3 **Portion Control:**

- Be mindful of portion sizes to prevent overeating. Use measuring tools or visualize recommended serving sizes to maintain calorie control.
- Focus on the quality of your food choices rather than relying solely on quantity.

4 **Smart Snacking:**

- Choose healthy snacks such as fresh fruits, nuts, or yogurt to curb hunger between meals.
- Avoid processed snacks high in sodium, saturated fats, and added sugars.

5 Consistent Hydration:

- Drink an adequate amount of water throughout the day to support overall health and assist in maintaining proper hydration levels.

6 Regular Exercise:

- Complement your dietary efforts with regular physical activity, as recommended by your healthcare provider.
- Mix up your regimen by including strength training, flexibility training, and cardiovascular workouts.

7 Tracking Progress:

- Keep a food journal or use a mobile app to track your meals, snacks, and water intake.
- Monitor any changes in your health metrics, such as blood pressure, to assess the impact of the DASH diet.

8 Social Support:

- Share your commitment to the DASH diet with friends or family, fostering a supportive environment.

- Engage in activities that align with your dietary goals, making it easier to stay on track during social gatherings.

9 Educational Resources:

- Continuously educate yourself about the DASH diet through reputable sources, staying informed about its benefits and the latest research.

10 Mindful Eating Practices:

- Savor each bite, be aware of your body's signals of hunger and fullness, and keep your eyes off other things as you eat to cultivate mindful eating.

Overcoming Challenges

Successfully navigating challenges while utilizing the Complete DASH Diet Cookbook for Beginners involves a comprehensive strategy. Below, I'll delve into specific aspects to address potential hurdles and enhance your experience with the DASH diet.

1 Understanding DASH Principles:

Begin by thoroughly understanding the principles of the DASH diet, which focuses on reducing sodium intake, emphasizing whole foods, and promoting nutrient-rich choices. Familiarize yourself with the recommended servings of various food groups.

2 Equipping Your Kitchen:

Ensure your kitchen is well-equipped with tools and ingredients essential for DASH-friendly cooking. This includes herbs, spices, whole grains, lean proteins, and a variety of fruits and vegetables.

3 Tackling Taste Concerns:

Experiment with herbs and spices to add flavor without relying on excessive salt. Explore healthy flavor enhancers like garlic, lemon, and vinegar. Utilize cooking techniques such as roasting, grilling, and sautéing to bring out natural flavors.

4 Diversifying Cooking Methods:

Combat monotony by diversifying your cooking methods. Incorporate raw, steamed, and grilled options to maintain variety in textures and flavors, making your meals more enjoyable.

5 Effective Meal Planning:

Overcome the challenge of maintaining a balanced diet with effective meal planning. Create a weekly menu that aligns with DASH guidelines. This not only streamlines grocery shopping but also ensures a well-rounded, nutritious intake.

6 Time Management:

Address time constraints by embracing efficient cooking practices. Consider batch cooking and meal prepping to save time on busy days. Cook larger portions and freeze individual servings for quick, DASH-compliant meals.

7 Social Situations:

Navigate social situations by communicating your dietary needs to friends and family. Offer to contribute a DASH-friendly dish when attending gatherings to ensure there's a healthy option available for you.

8 Motivation and Goal Setting:

Stay motivated by setting realistic, achievable goals. Track your progress and celebrate small victories. Regularly reassess your goals, making adjustments as needed to keep your journey with the DASH diet dynamic and sustainable.

9 Support Networks:

Connect with online communities, friends, or family members who are also following the DASH diet. Exchanges of tales, techniques, and advice may be quite energizing and supportive.

10 Mindful Eating:

Overcome challenges by practicing mindful eating. Savor every bite and pay heed to your body's signals of hunger and fullness. This can help you make conscious food choices aligned with the DASH principles.

Incorporating DASH Principles Long-Term

Incorporating DASH (Dietary Approaches to Stop Hypertension) principles into your lifestyle for the long term involves making sustainable changes to your dietary habits. The DASH diet is renowned for its effectiveness in managing blood pressure and promoting heart health. Here's an extensive guide on how to seamlessly integrate DASH principles into your daily life for lasting benefits:

1. Educate Yourself:
>   Understand the core principles of the DASH diet, emphasizing the importance of reducing sodium intake, increasing nutrient-rich foods, and maintaining a balanced diet.

2. Assess Current Eating Habits:
>   Evaluate your current dietary habits to identify areas that need adjustment. Recognize patterns of high sodium intake and prioritize areas for improvement.

3. Set Realistic Goals:
>   Establish achievable, realistic goals to implement DASH principles. Gradual changes are more likely to become lasting

habits compared to drastic, unsustainable modifications.

4. Emphasize Fruits and Vegetables:

Increase the variety and quantity of fruits and vegetables in your diet. Aim for a colorful mix, as different hues indicate diverse nutrient profiles.

5. Whole Grains Over Refined Grains:

Transition from refined grains to whole grains. Incorporate options like brown rice, quinoa, whole wheat pasta, and oats to enhance fiber intake.

6. Prioritize Lean Proteins:

Choose lean protein sources such as poultry, fish, legumes, and tofu. Limit red meat consumption and opt for healthier protein alternatives.

7. Mindful Sodium Reduction:

Gradually reduce your sodium intake by using herbs, spices, and other flavorings to season your food. Be cautious with processed and packaged foods, as they often contain high levels of sodium.

8. Healthy Fats:

Include foods like avocados, almonds, seeds, and olive oil in your diet as sources of healthful fats. These fats support overall heart health.

9. Low-Fat Dairy Options:

Choose low-fat or fat-free dairy products to meet calcium needs while minimizing saturated fat intake. Incorporate alternatives like almond or soy milk if dairy isn't your preference.

10. Hydration:

Prioritize water consumption to stay adequately hydrated. Limit sugary beverages and alcohol, as excessive intake can have negative effects on blood pressure.

11. Cooking at Home:

Cook more meals at home to have better control over ingredients and preparation methods. This allows you to experiment with DASH-friendly recipes.

13. Monitor Sodium in Packaged Foods:

Read food labels to identify and monitor sodium content in packaged items. Choose low-sodium or sodium-free alternatives whenever possible.

14. Regular Check-Ins:

Schedule regular check-ins with healthcare professionals to monitor your blood pressure and assess the impact of DASH principles on your overall health.

15. Lifestyle Integration:

View DASH as a lifestyle rather than a temporary fix. Embrace it as a holistic approach to well-being, encompassing not only dietary choices but also stress management, regular physical activity, and adequate sleep.

16. Seek Support:

Share your DASH journey with friends or family members. Having a support system can make it easier to maintain long-term adherence to healthier eating habits.

FITNESS AND LIFESTYLE TIPS

Exercise Recommendations

Incorporating exercise into your routine while following the DASH (Dietary Approaches to Stop Hypertension) diet is crucial for overall health. Here are comprehensive exercise recommendations to complement the DASH diet in the Complete DASH Diet Cookbook for Beginners:

1 **Cardiovascular Exercise (Aerobic):**

- Try to get in at least 150 minutes a week of moderate-to-intense aerobic activity, such swimming, cycling, or brisk walking.
- Include activities that elevate your heart rate, promoting cardiovascular health and aiding in weight management.

2 **Strength Training:**

- Integrate strength training exercises at least twice a week to build and maintain muscle mass.

- Incorporate bodyweight exercises, resistance bands, or free weights to target major muscle groups.

3 Flexibility and Stretching:

- Allocate time for stretching exercises to enhance flexibility and reduce the risk of injuries.
- Yoga or Pilates can be excellent choices, helping to improve balance and posture.

4 Interval Training:

- Introduce interval training to boost metabolism and enhance cardiovascular fitness.
- Alternating between high-intensity bursts and periods of lower intensity can be effective for burning calories.

5 Incorporate Daily Activity:

- Include more physical activity in your daily routine, such as taking stairs, walking instead of driving for short distances, or gardening.
- Aim for a minimum of 10,000 steps per day to promote overall well-being.

6 Consistency is Key:

- Create a sustainable exercise routine that aligns with your lifestyle and preferences.
- Consistency is crucial for long-term health benefits, so find activities you enjoy and make them a regular part of your schedule.

7 Consult with a Professional:

- Before starting any new exercise program, especially if you have underlying health conditions, consult with a healthcare professional or a certified fitness expert.

8 Hydration and Recovery:

- Stay well-hydrated during exercise, and prioritize post-workout recovery with proper nutrition and rest.
- Adequate recovery is essential for muscle repair and overall well-being.

9 Listen to Your Body:

- Pay attention to your body's signals. If you experience pain or discomfort, modify your exercise routine and seek guidance from a healthcare professional.

10 Progress Tracking:

- Keep track of your fitness progress to stay motivated and make necessary adjustments to your routine.

Stress Management

Stress management is crucial for maintaining overall well-being, and incorporating it into a comprehensive approach like the DASH (Dietary Approaches to Stop Hypertension) diet can enhance its effectiveness. The DASH diet emphasizes nutrient-rich foods and has been linked to various health benefits, including stress reduction.

1. **Balanced Nutrition:** The DASH diet encourages the consumption of fruits, vegetables, whole grains, lean proteins, and low-fat dairy products. These foods provide essential nutrients that support overall mental and physical health. Adequate intake of vitamins and minerals, such as B-vitamins, magnesium, and antioxidants, can positively impact stress levels.

2. **Omega-3 Fatty Acids:** The DASH diet promotes the consumption of fatty fish, nuts,

and seeds, which are rich in omega-3 fatty acids. These fatty acids have been associated with reducing symptoms of stress and anxiety. Including sources of omega-3s in your diet can contribute to better stress management.

3. **Hydration:** Proper hydration is essential for overall health, including mental well-being. The DASH diet encourages water intake and discourages excessive consumption of sugary beverages, which can impact mood and energy levels. Staying adequately hydrated is a simple yet effective way to support stress management.

4. **Mindful Eating Practices:** Incorporate mindfulness into your meals by savoring each bite, paying attention to flavors and textures. Mindful eating has been shown to reduce stress by promoting a healthier relationship with food. The DASH diet, with its focus on whole and unprocessed foods, aligns well with mindful eating principles.

5. **Meal Planning and Preparation:** The DASH diet cookbook for beginners can guide individuals in planning and preparing balanced meals. Having a well-organized meal plan reduces the stress associated

with last-minute decisions and ensures a
consistent intake of nutritious foods.

6. **Limiting Processed Foods and Sodium:**
   High intake of processed foods and
   excessive sodium can contribute to stress
   and negatively impact overall health. The
   DASH diet recommends minimizing
   processed and high-sodium foods,
   promoting a diet that supports
   cardiovascular health and stress reduction.

7. **Social Connection and Support:** The
   DASH diet can be more enjoyable when
   shared with others. Connecting with friends
   or family for shared meals and mutual
   support can enhance the positive impact of
   both the diet and stress management
   efforts.

8. **Physical Activity:** While not directly related
   to the DASH diet cookbook, incorporating
   regular physical activity is a key component
   of stress management. The DASH diet can
   complement an active lifestyle, contributing
   to overall health and well-being.

7 DAYS SAMPLE WEEKLY MEAL PLAN

Day	Breakfast	Lunch	Dinner	snacks
Day 1	Greek yogurt parfait with fresh berries and a sprinkle of nuts. Whole grain toast with avocado.	Grilled chicken salad with mixed greens, cherry tomatoes, cucumbers, and a light olive oil dressing. Quinoa or brown rice on the side.	Baked salmon with lemon and herbs. Steamed broccoli and carrots. Mashed sweet potatoes.	Apple slices with a tablespoon of almond butter.

Day				
Day 2	Oatmeal topped with sliced bananas and a drizzle of honey. Low-fat milk or a dairy-free alternative	Turkey and vegetable wrap with whole grain tortilla. Mixed fruit salad	Stir-fried tofu with mixed vegetables.	Carrot and celery sticks with hummus.
Day 3	Spinach and feta omelette. Whole grain English muffin.	Lentil soup with a side of whole grain crackers Mixed green salad with a balsamic vinaigrette	Grilled shrimp with a lemon and garlic marinade Roasted Brussels sprouts Wild rice	Handful of unsalted nuts

| Day 4 | Smoothie with spinach, banana, berries, and low-fat yogurt

Whole grain toast with peanut butter | Quinoa salad with chickpeas, cherry tomatoes, and feta cheese

Whole grain roll | Baked chicken breast with rosemary and thyme

Steamed green beans

Quinoa or brown rice | Orange slices |
|---|---|---|---|---|
| Day 5 | Whole grain oatmeal with berries.

Overnight Oatmeal | Warm Rice & Pintos Salad

Lentil soup with a side of mixed greens. | Baked salmon, quinoa, and steamed broccoli.

Turkey meatb | Lemon-Blueberry Muffins |

			alls, whole wheat pasta, and marinara sauce.	
Day 6	Greek yogurt with sliced banana.	Quinoa and black bean bowl with salsa. Chickpea salad wrap with whole grain tortilla.	Stir-fried tofu with vegetables and brown rice. Grilled shrimp skewers, quinoa, and roasted asparagus. Layered Vegetable	Raspberry Peach Puff Pancake

			Salad	
Day **7**	Smoothie with spinach, banana, and almond milk.	Quinoa and vegetable stir-fry. Grilled Southwestern Steak Salad	Baked cod with sweet potato wedges and green beans. Tuna Salad (as a sandwich or on its own) Cabbage Roll Skillet	Lemon-Blueberry Muffins

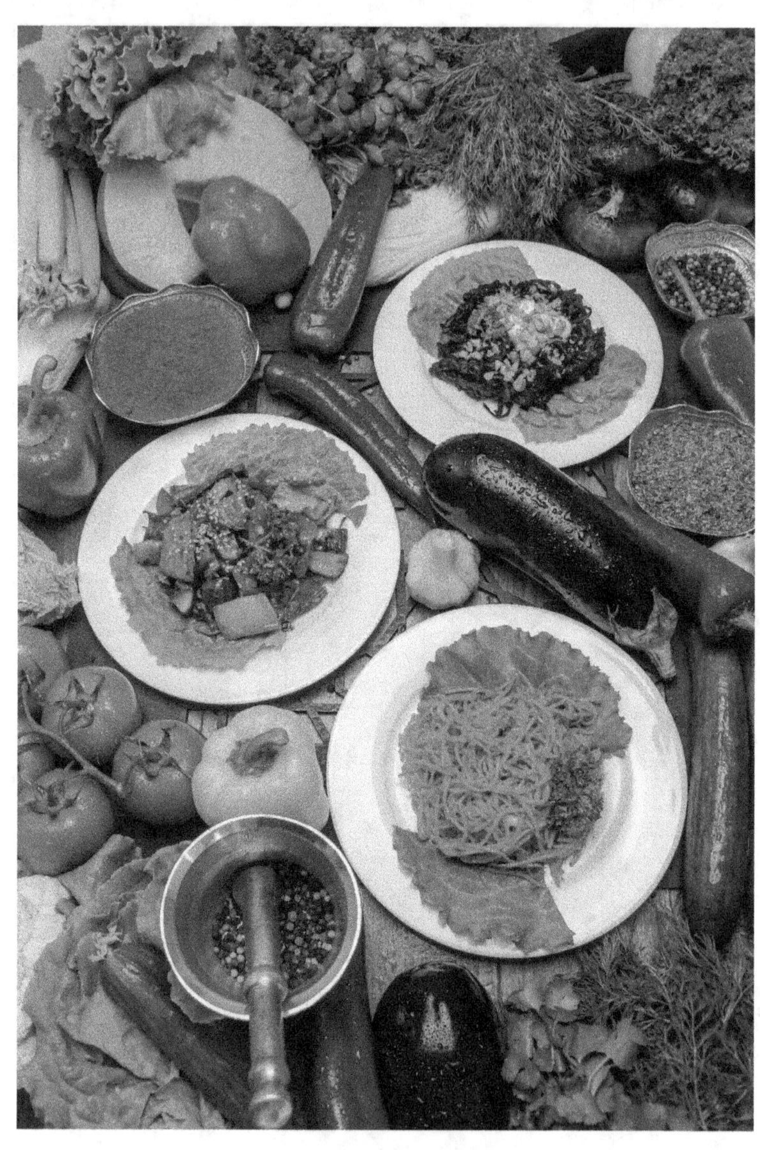

CONCLUSION

The Complete DASH Diet Cookbook for Beginners offers more than just a compilation of recipes; it serves as a comprehensive guide to transforming your eating habits and, consequently, your overall well-being. As you reach the end of this culinary journey, it's crucial to reflect on the multifaceted benefits this cookbook brings to your life.

First and foremost, the diverse range of recipes presented here ensures that adopting the DASH diet is not a restrictive chore but a flavorful adventure. From breakfast to dinner and snacks in between, the cookbook provides an extensive array of delicious options that align with the principles of the DASH diet. This variety not only keeps your taste buds engaged but also makes the transition to a heart-healthy lifestyle enjoyable.

Moreover, the cookbook doesn't merely focus on the what but delves into the why. The educational components scattered throughout the pages empower you with the knowledge needed to make informed choices about your diet. Understanding the science behind the DASH diet gives you a deeper appreciation for the positive impact each meal can have on your cardiovascular health. This knowledge becomes a powerful tool in your journey towards sustained well-being.

Beyond the recipes and educational insights, this cookbook serves as a practical resource. It provides meal plans, shopping lists, and cooking tips, streamlining the process of incorporating DASH principles into your daily life. The user-friendly approach ensures that even beginners can seamlessly integrate these healthful practices into their routine.

In essence, the Complete DASH Diet Cookbook for Beginners is a holistic companion on your path to better health. It's not just about the food you put on your plate; it's about cultivating a mindful and balanced relationship with what you eat. As you conclude this culinary exploration, relish in the fact that you've not only expanded your recipe repertoire but also taken significant steps towards prioritizing your heart health. This cookbook is an investment in your long-term well-being, and with each meal, you're contributing to a healthier, happier you. Cheers to savoring both the flavors and the benefits of the DASH diet!